Nutrition For Beginners

Increase Your Health, Increase your Lifespan

By: Tammy Jones

Table of Contents

Introduction

This book contains proven steps and strategies on how to feed yourself better. It is clear that not eating enough food or eating foods that are too rich in fat or sugar can be very harmful to your body.

For most of us, we are not aware that the body needs a certain quantity and quality of nutrients every day in order to function normally that's mostly because we live in a world where fast and easy foods that are most of the time highly processed are aggressively marketed. Overall, what is important to remember here is that when you eat too much of foods that are poor in the vital nutrients your body will end up having a harder time processing it, leading to more unhealthy fat retention and other complications in the long run. You'll have to train yourself to eat better (healthier) so that you just get enough daily nutrients to stay healthy and most of all, sustain a healthy weight.

I hope you enjoy it!

Chapter 1-What Is Good Nutrition?

Nutrition has always been an issue, and the food industry is somehow to blame for it. It is now well-known that additives such as maple syrup are added to most processed food in order to make them taste better, hence adding too much sugar to food just to make it more appealing to people's tastes. If their consumption (processed foods) is not regulated or accompanied by regular physical exercises, then people end up lacking the proper nutrients they need for their body to function, and it can also lead to weight gain and obesity. So, in this chapter, we will cover what is generally seen as good nutrition, which is the one that helps you stay healthy and maintain a healthy weight throughout your life.

What should your body absorb every day in terms of calories?

There is a certain number of calories that a human being needs to ingest every day in order to have a functioning body, be healthy, and maintain a healthy body weight. The normal intake of calories for women is 2000 calories in order to maintain a healthy weight. And for men, 2,500 calories to maintain a healthy weight. Of course, all of this works with regular exercise and good nutrition.

What types of nutrients are recommended every day?

Normally, anything natural needs to be prioritized here (and preferably organic because of the GMO issue). One will ask, but what about snacks that are highly processed? It would be naïve to think that someone wouldn't eat a bar of chocolate or grab a bag of chips from time to time, but when eaten excessively during the day or during long periods of time, they become substitutes to the food you are normally supposed to ingest every day, and they normally cause problems because the body cannot process them in the long run and they can also lead to certain diseases (like obesity and certain cancers).

So, foodstuff like fruits, vegetables, and certain meats are mostly recommended.

So, this is what you should remember overall, the body needs a certain intake of healthy fats (like fatty acids for your brain's health), enough vitamins (A,B,C,D, etc.), protein (mostly found in meats), Calcium (for your bones), Potassium, iron (for your blood) and foods rich in antioxidants (that help your body heal faster). Let's now go through a list of what these nutrients bring to your body:

Protein: This is probably the most necessary and most important nutrient of them all, because all of your organs need protein to function every day. Protein is often found in red meat and white meat. But you should also eat meat moderately, and perhaps alternate meat with other types of food that are rich in protein as well, like eggs or broccoli.

Fatty or Omega 3 Acids: They are generally found in nuts or in certain oily fish like salmon. Foods that are rich in fatty acids are known to help fight conditions like rheumatoid arthritis, depression (it is known to help soothe the effects of antidepressants) and also helps babies develop better while still in their mother's womb (they are known to help with visual and neurological development in infants.)

Calcium: Calcium is a mineral necessary for building bones and keeping them healthy. Added to its benefits, you can also count enabling our blood to clot, proper muscle contraction, and also enabling our heart to beat at a normal rate. It is found in food stuffs like milk and other dairy products.

Potassium: It is a mineral and at the same time an electrolyte. It is good for muscles and is mostly found in foods like apricots, prunes, raisins, orange juice, bananas, etc.

Vitamins: Known as an organic molecule, it is essential for the organism but in small quantities, mostly for the proper functioning of its metabolism. Overall, there are about 13 known types of vitamins.

Iron: You'll find iron in foodstuff like spinach and dark chocolate. Iron is an essential nutrient that helps bring oxygen to our blood and it is also responsible for the production of energy in our whole body. You can also find it in foodstuffs like beans, lentils, tofu, baked potatoes, dark leafy vegetables, and cashew just to name a few.

Antioxidants: Antioxidants as said earlier, help our body fight infections, heart diseases, and also prevent you from developing certain cancers. Examples of foods that are rich in antioxidants are blueberries, blue grapes, nuts, dark green veggies, sweet potatoes, and carrots (and other orange vegetables).

This is more or less the types of foods you should look for if you want to have a balanced diet and stay healthy. Let's now see how you can organize your meals every day, following all the guidelines we've covered so far.

How to organize your plate/meals every day and still get the right nutrients?

When it comes to getting the right nutrients every day, meaning just getting a bit of everything every day, the key is to do the following (or if you prefer, to have the reflexes below):

- First, you have to think of spreading your list of essential nutrients throughout the day, meaning that you should make sure you have enough protein, antioxidants, iron, vitamins, Potassium, calcium, and fatty acids in your diet. That's why it is always good to get enough information about the types of food you bring into your house. That is because many foodstuffs can contain 2, 3 or more nutrients at once, out of all the ones we've listed in our previous section. Examples of such food are kale (which is rich in vitamins C, A, and K1), seaweed (rich in Calcium, iron, magnesium, and antioxidants), Shellfish (which is rich in various B vitamins, Potassium, Selenium, and Iron), potatoes (rich in Potassium, Magnesium, Iron, Copper, and

Magnesium), and liver (rich in Vitamins B12, B5, B6, B2, A, Copper, Selenium, and animal Protein.)

- Next, take into consideration the number of calories you should ingest per day with regards to your gender (2000 for women, 2,500 for men.)

- Decide how many meals you want to have per day, which is normally 4 meals per day (with breakfast, lunch, an afternoon snack, and later on, dinner).

- Evaluate the importance of meals with respect to calorie intake. Meaning that Your breakfast should have the most calories, followed by lunch, snacks, and dinner (should have the least calories). And the total should not exceed 2000 (for women) or 2,500 (for men).

- Then, organize your plate per meal. Remember the rule is to maximize the number of vegetables or fruits, get a little bit of meat and then a little bit of starch on the side. So, if the plate represents 100%, vegetables should take 50% of the plate area, the meat 25% of the plate area, and the starch (rice, fries, potatoes) also 25% of your plate area.

So, overall, eating well means eating healthy enough and also getting the right information out there. And also, remember that healthy food doesn't mean less taste than your favorite burger or French fries, you just have to learn to cook for yourself a bit more and put a little bit of willpower when it comes to it.

What to retain from this Chapter:
- Good nutrition is about ingesting the right nutrients on a daily basis.

- You have to know what you put on your plate, so information about the food that is available out there is important.

- Taking into consideration the recommended number of calories that one should ingest every day is essential to maintaining a healthy weight.

- Some foods out there are rich in various nutrients and should form part of your diet from now on.

Chapter 2-Nutrition for Active People

Throughout this book, you will see that we will cover many ways to feed yourself, which are also linked to how active you are every day, in other words to your lifestyle. That's mostly because if you are active you might want to feed and also hydrate yourself more, in order to recover the water you've lost while working out and also feed your body with the most energetic foodstuff that is available and healthy for you. Let's now cover ways to help you keep a healthy and balancing diet all by also being active.

What Nutrients do you need as an active person?

It is clear that added to their normal diets, active people (those who work out a lot) need nutrients that will help them grow stronger, build muscles, replace the water they've just lost while exercising, and, of course, have enough energy for the rest of the day. So, your main goals here would be to energize your body as much as you can, repairing or building muscles, fortify your bones, and of course drink lots of water. This is what you should look forward to (in terms of foods) in order to achieve these goals:

- For energy eat lots of grains, notably by consuming bread, pasta, oatmeal, cereals, and tortillas.

- For muscle repair or build up, eat lean or low-fat cuts of meats like beef or pork. You'll also have to consume chicken with no skin (chicken breasts), turkey and lots of seafood.

- Drink lots of water, between 8 to 10 cups a day. Go for filtered or purified water to minimize toxins and other harmful bacteria.

- And, of course, eat lots of vegetables and fruits, which are also great sources of plant protein. The trick is to choose as many colors of fruits there is out there (as each color hides a specific beneficial nutrient like, for instance, orange fruits which are rich in carotene which works great for the skin).

- Also, you should diminish your intake in sugary and high sodium foods by picking from frozen low sodium canned, dried or 100% juice (not syrup) option.

How many calories should you ingest per day?

For people who are active, maintaining an ideal lean body or a certain weight is ideal, then your calorie intake should be slightly slower than the average man or woman. So, if, for instance, a non-active woman ingests 2,000 calories a day, an active one should ingest less, which is 1,500 calories. For men, the same applies, where for non-active ones 2,500 calories are recommended and for active ones, they should ingest less with a recommended 2,000 calories a day. One would ask why the difference? Well, it's simple. If you've started working out, you would want to see results fast or reach your goals after a certain period of time, so lowering your caloric intake does help you lose weight faster and better enables you to adopt an active life, with less weight and certainly more energy to work out every day.

How many times a day should you eat when being an active person?

Well, since you are supposed to work out, people would expect you to eat more. Which is not necessarily true because you still have to maintain a lean and healthy body. So, your 4 meals are required, just like ordinary people. You are also recommended to eat in the morning right after working out and not before it (simply because you might jeopardize your workout session by throwing up the food or being uncomfortable). Breakfast is the most important meal, and arranging your calorie intake making sure breakfast has the most out of the 1,500 (for women) and 2,000 (for men) , then dinner with the second most calories (so that you wake up energized to get back at working out in the morning), and then lunch and snacks with the third and fourth least calorie intake of the day.

Once again, use the plate technique to measure the nutrients you put in your body. This time include grains (or foodstuff made out of grains), fruits and veggies, and protein. Where protein makes up 25% of your plate, grains 25% of your plate area, and fruits and vegetables 50% of your plate area (25/25).

One last thing that we would like to add is the use of liquids throughout the day. You should always drink 8 to 10 glasses for hydration purposes and the elimination of toxins (too much toxins can also lead to gain weight in the long run). And if you have cravings during the day, you can add 1 to 2 smoothies during the day to your regular diet, with fruits and vegetables making part of it (without sugar added to them). Liquified fruits and vegetables are easier to digest for the body and are richer with essential nutrients, which will help with your cravings without necessarily leading to gain weight.

What to retain in this chapter:

- Active people should consume fewer calories than ordinary ones

- Active people have 2 main meals which are breakfast and dinner (respectively).

- The use of liquids and liquified foods are essential for active people because it helps get rid of cravings and are easy to digest as well.

Chapter 3-Superfoods for the Sceptics

Superfoods are groups of foods that we often neglect or totally ignore but that give us more essential daily nutrients than the food we are already used to. To better learn about them you will obviously have to know what they are, and then pick the ones you believe will suit your diet best (or that you feel you can easily introduce in your diet.)

What are superfoods?

The term "superfood" is something we seem to be hearing and reading about almost every day. It serves to describe a group of foods that are packed with healthy nutrients that can help us feed ourselves but also prevent or cure certain conditions (mostly cancers, heart diseases, and even depression.) Some specialists would say that there's nothing special about them and that it might just be a marketing stunt coming from the food industry, but for most skeptics, who don't know how to feed themselves, or who don't know who to ask about a better nutritional plan for themselves, giving it a try will not be disappointing, and it is mostly because these specific foods have the power to feed you but also to heel you (to some extent).

How to know the ones that are good for you?

The only way to answer this question, because, we believe that's what a skeptic would ask right away, is to look at what each of them has to offer, is to ask yourself, "are they going to keep me away from certain infections?", "Will I be able to avoid cancers, low blood pressure, and other diseases after consuming them for a long time?", "can they easily get molded into my habits or lifestyle?", and, "are they culinarily flexible?" (or, if you prefer, are they easy to cook or great supplements?). So, after doing your research about some of them (because you won't be able to cover them all in a short period of time), make a list, and narrow this list down to those who answer to these specific questions.

Here, is below a list of examples of superfoods, just to let you see what they are capable to bring to your diet:

- Dark green leafy vegetables, like kale, swiss chard, collard greens, turnip greens, and spinach. They are renown for being excellent sources of nutrients like folate, zinc, calcium, iron, magnesium, vitamin C, fiber, and high levels of anti-inflammatory compounds known as carotenoids, which are known to protect against certain types of cancer.

- Berries, such as raspberries, strawberries, blueberries, blackberries, cranberries. They are all known to be a nutritional powerhouse of minerals, fiber, vitamins, and antioxidants. They are all high in antioxidants which can help prevent conditions such as heart diseases, cancers, and other inflammatory diseases.

- Green Tea, which is originally from China. It is renowned to be rich in antioxidants and polyphenolic compounds which are known to have strong anti-inflammatory effects on the body.

- Eggs, although reputed to be high in cholesterol, they also contain many nutrients like B vitamins, choline, selenium, vitamin A, iron, phosperous and are also loaded with high-quality protein. Eggs contain 2 antioxidants known as zeaxanthin and lutein, which are known to protect eye health and vision.

- Legumes, such as beans, lentils, peas, peanuts, and falafel. They are known to be a class of plant foods rich in B Vitamins, minerals, protein and fiber. They are known to help improve type 2 diabetes, to reduce blood pressure and cholesterol.

- Nuts and seeds, such as almonds, peanuts, sunflower seeds, pumpkin seeds, chia seeds, and hemp seeds.)

Nuts and seeds are known to be rich in fiber, vegetarian protein, and heart-healthy fats. Added to these, they also contain plant compounds with anti-inflammatory and antioxidants properties that can effectively protect against oxidative stress.

This list contains a list of superfoods that you might already be familiar with but didn't know they have all the properties quoted above. There are more superfoods out there, and to get a more extensive list, for those of you who are curious about getting more options speak to your local dietician about wanting to insert them into your diets from now on.

How to incorporate them into your diet?

The most effective way to incorporate them into your diet is to use them as supplements (as foodstuff that you can use to replace other's that you normally eat but are less healthy), and also revise your list of snacks during the day, so that they can be completely replaced by one of the known superfoods. Make sure that, in order to see their effects, you make the swap (for ordinary food to superfoods) for a long period of time, so that you take advantage of their benefits for longer.

What to retain from this chapter:

- Superfoods have a very diverse and high nutritional value, in general.

- Superfoods work best when treated like supplements, complements, or replacements for ordinary but less rich foodstuff.

- Superfoods, when consumed over long periods of time, can help reverse certain conditions or diseases.

Chapter 4-Nutrition for Pregnant Women

Pregnant women need to feed themselves better as well, for obvious reasons they have more than enough reasons to ingest the right nutrients for their babies and themselves. It might be very delicate because pregnant women are more tempted to eat anything and everything all day and all night long. Well, there's a way to help them eat what they need and in the right quantity.

What do you really need while pregnant?

It is clear and always recommended to get the appropriate nutrients and energy while pregnant for you and your baby's health. That's why the use of vitamins containing iron, calcium, fatty acids, and other minerals are important added to that, pregnant women should at least take 400 mg a day of folic acid. You must also make sure that all your meals contain enough protein (so eat meat and plants that are rich in protein), carbohydrates, fats, vitamins, and minerals. And, since you are eating for two, make sure that your calorie intake is 300 more per day (this is to help the baby grow normally) than what you regularly get. Meaning that if you were ingesting 2,000 calories every day before pregnancy, your calorie intake during pregnancy should be 2,300 every day.

Now, although you can eat anything you can as long as it has the right nutrients there are also things you cannot eat while pregnant because it could damage the baby's health. These types of foods comprise:

- Meats that are raw like uncooked seafood and rare uncooked beef or poultry. Because they could lead to salmonella infection, toxoplasmosis, and also the risks of contamination with coliform bacteria.

- Deli meat which could cause miscarriages because of the risks of Listeria contamination.

- Certain fish like shark, swordfish, king mackerel and tilefish, which are high in mercury and if consumed could lead to developmental delays and even brain damage for the baby, while pregnant.

- Smoked seafood like refrigerated lox, nova styled or kippered smoked seafood, because of risks of Listeria contamination.

- Raw shellfish like oysters, clams, and mussels should also be avoided.

- Certain homemade recipes like homemade ice cream, custards, mayonnaise, etc., because of the potential exposure to salmonella.

- Soft cheese, as well as unpasteurized milk, should be avoided while pregnant because of the potential risks of Listeria. Avoid most of all, imported soft cheeses like brie, camembert, Roquefort, feta, Gorgonzola, and Mexican style cheeses.

- Avoid pate or meat spread as well because they also contain the bacteria Listeria.

- Caffeine should be avoided during the first trimester since it has been proven to be linked to certain miscarriages.

- Alcohol consumed during pregnancy could lead to developmental disorders in the child, so it should be avoided at all costs.

How many times should you eat while pregnant?

Pregnant women seem to be hungry all the time, so, meal restriction is normally not recommended because cravings are often common with them. However, in order to avoid certain conditions with the baby and yourself during and after pregnancy, you should make sure that you not only eat healthily but that your daily meals respect the 2,300-calorie intake that is recommended. So, avoid too much-processed foods as much as you can, and eat washed fruits and veggies as well as cooked healthy meals that can be processed by your body. Eat as many fruits as you can for breakfast, and consistent, but preferably home cooked meals for lunch and dinner. Consider your cravings like the potential opportunity to eat snacks and indulge in healthy and natural foods that are low in calories.

What to retain for this chapter:

- Although there are no restrictions on what you should eat during pregnancy, you should only add 300 calories in your daily diet every day.

- You should watch what you eat while pregnant because not all foods are good for the baby and could lead to certain contaminations.

- Although there are no limitations into the number of times a pregnant woman should eat, eating consistent meals during the day, could help you respect the 2,300 calories intake that is normally recommended for pregnant women.

Chapter 5-Nutrition for the Busy Ones

It is also important to address busy people's nutrition because busy people almost never have the time to feed themselves the right way. They are the ones who are more exposed to junk food and malnourishment (with not enough nutrients or food with too much sugar and fat.)

There are ways to get what you need from food even during your busiest days.

Although busy people seem to be often taken by time and never seem to have enough time for themselves, they still need their 1,500 to 2,000 calorie intake a day for women or 2,000 to 2,500 calorie intake for men a day. And as long as eating doesn't make them want to sleep and waste time, they should be okay. So, here, food supplements are necessary during each meal. You can eat your normal 4 meals for the day, but this time around, you should focus on foods that give you energy like bran cereals in the morning and certain foods like bananas and apples, plus coffee or tea (plus your recommended dose of morning vitamins), proceed the same way to lunch, with a salad or a meat sandwich with only natural ingredients and water (plus your daily intake of supplements or vitamins). At night you may not need any supplements, but make sure you eat a consistent meal that can fill you up, but also lead you to sleep with ease (turkey, rice, beans are often recommended for that purpose.)

Avoid processed, sugary foods at night because of their risks of keeping you awake and excited and you should also avoid drinking more than 2 cups of coffee per day. Make sure you avoid drinking coffee after 5 pm because of the risks of insomnia that it may lead to. Make time (20 to 25 minutes) to eat and digest your meals and favor water to anything else as your choice of drink after a meal, especially after breakfast.

How can you eat right and at the same time manage a busy schedule?

Managing a schedule isn't that difficult if you have the right tools and reflexes to set everything up. Once you've set up your plan to go with, all that is left to do is apply it. When it comes to regulating how you eat every day it's simple, even though many people choose to omit it, simply find an appropriate spot in your schedule for your 3 meals that occur during the most important period of the day, which is breakfast in the morning, and then, find 2 more spots in your schedule, where you can spend eating your meals or snacks for 20 to 25 minutes.

Another thing that you should look at is planning in advance on what you should eat while outside taking care of business. It is better and easier to know what is recommended for you to eat while in the rush and in need of a proper meal. Look for items like meat sandwiches with natural ingredients, salads, certain low-fat dairies, grains, fruits, certain smoothies, and of course, low-fat processed or unprocessed foods.

What to retain from this chapter:

- Being busy doesn't mean putting your normal everyday nutrition under jeopardy.

- Insert your mealtimes into your schedule.

- Indulge in energy packed nutrients in the morning.

- Eat light meals during the day but eat consistently and healthily at night before sleep.

- Stick to 2 cups of coffee during the day and not more in order not to compromise the quality of your sleep.

Chapter 6-Nutrition for Those Who Are Dieting

Another important aspect that should be covered is dieting. Many people diet to lose weight, and when they say losing weight, they mean losing weight at all costs. So, if a certain diet is incompatible for whatever reason or deemed too aggressive, one might end up gaining all the weight back or missing some important nutrients.

So, we will now cover a few important points someone should have in mind when dieting.

What type of nutrients one should focus on when dieting?

Some studies conducted at the Harvard University has concluded that foods rich in protein (like red meat), certain starches (like rice, pasta, potatoes), dietary foods (like certain butters), should be consumed sparingly (rarely), and are actually put at the top of the healthy eating pyramid (which makes them the least healthy of all foods). Next, come dairy or calcium supplements that should be consumed once or twice a day, followed by fish, poultry, and eggs that should either be suppressed or eaten at least twice a day. Then, come the healthiest options which are nuts and dried fruits followed by fruits and vegetables that are recommended to eat at most 3 times a day. The most recommended eating/healthy habits when dieting, according to their healthy eating pyramid would be to consume whole grain foods, healthy oils from plants and of course, exercise a lot. This, overall, sums up what you should focus or prioritize on when you decide to go on a diet. Now, in our previous chapters, we've focused more on the nutrients that were important when wanting to feed yourself better. In this chapter, we will now explain why some groups of foods should be favored a little bit more than others.

- Protein shouldn't be cut off your diet because it is the main food source that gives you energy and keeps you going during the day. You have to remember that it is not only meats that contain protein, you have a long list of plants and vegetables that are also high in protein (see chapter 1 for more details).

- Fats are also important, but the good ones found in salmon fish also known as omega 3s fats. It is because they help protect your brain and heart.

- Fiber should also be kept in your diet while dieting. You should eat grains, fruits, vegetables, nuts, and beans to get your daily intake of fiber. They will help you stay regular (helping with digestion) but also help you lower risks of heart diseases, stroke, and diabetes. They can also help improve your skin and lose weight.

- Calcium, not only does it help you fight osteoporosis, but it also helps fight anxiety, depression, and sleep difficulties. Eating foods that are rich in magnesium, vitamins D and K are also important because they help the body absorb calcium even better, which is good to know.

- And lastly, Carbohydrates which also help your body store up energy during the day. You should get most of it in complex and unrefined carbs like vegetables, whole grains, and fruits) rather than sugars and refined carbs.

To sum it all up what you should cut back on while dieting is highly processed foods like white bread, pastries, starches, and sugar.

How many times someone should eat while dieting?

When you diet, you can still follow the 3 meals a day rule, but this time around, most of your nutrient filled foods should be eaten during breakfast, which should be the most consistent one of the day, followed by 3 other (smaller) meals during the day.

Remember to ingest 1,500 calories a day for women and 2,000 calories for men, and to also do the following:

- Eat your dinners earlier and make sure that there's a 14 to 16-hour gap between your last meal of the day and your next breakfast. Which makes it easier for your body to digest and process nutrients.

- Make breakfast the heaviest, but also the richest (in nutrients) meal of the day.

- Eat slowly and see food as a way to nourish yourself instead of a mean to satisfy your cravings for taste and flavors.

- Take your time to replace your choice of processed foods with healthier alternatives and stick with the change for good.

- Stop eating before or as soon as you feel full. This will prevent you from ingesting unwanted quantities if food, hence helping you to gain weight in the long run.

- Learn to read labels on your food packaging so you know what you are actually ingesting (look for calories and nutritional values).

- Before you eat something, think about how it will make you feel. Remember that healthy foods make you feel energized, while unhealthy ones make you feel drained out and unmotivated.

- And last but not least, drink plenty of water, because of its ability to help flush your systems of toxins (which in the long run can also lead to unwanted gain weight).

What type of diets works when you want to lose weight?

The right answer should be to follow a certain guideline that doesn't ask you to cut off important nutrients, but rather help you substitute your unhealthy habits with healthier alternatives. There are no magical diets that will help you lose weight because most of them ask you to cut off important nutritional sources. Instead follow these guidelines, while keeping in mind that all nutrients are essential to your body as long as they are natural (unprocessed):

- Eat in moderation, meaning that if you have to eat one serving of something stick to this one serving only. And also, try to alternate from one nutrient to another to bring some variety into your new diet.

- Also, reduce portion sizes on unhealthy foods gradually as you progress through your new weight-loss program.

- Think smaller portions. Sometimes we think with our eyes and fill up our plates leading us to eat more even when we are filled up.

- Take your time when you eat, meaning you shouldn't rush eating food that won't be fully crushed in your mouth and will, later on, be difficult for your body to process and distribute the nutrients your body needs for the day.

- Limit snacks during the day, especially processed ones. They may help you fight cravings during the day, but you can also get tempted to overindulge during the day, which can lead you to take bigger portions than you should. Limiting snacks can also help you fight emotional eating in the long run.

- Avoid eating late at night and keeping at least a 4-hour gap between meals during the day may help you regulate your weight even longer.

What to retain from this chapter:
- Knowing what should go into your plate while dieting is important.

- You shouldn't get rid of good nutrients because of the fear of gaining weight, instead, focus on natural and unprocessed food.

- Try to eat your dinner early at night in order to create a 14-hour gap between your last meal and your breakfast.

- When dieting, breakfast should be the most important meal of the day.

- Eat smaller portions of food during the day.

Conclusion

I hope this book was able to help you find ways to find an equilibrated diet that corresponds to your lifestyle. People often get it wrong when it comes to dieting because they believe that it's one diet, one recommendation, and one formula for everyone. They don't really look at your lifestyle, and certainly, don't think about the flexible aspect of a diet.

Hopefully, thanks to this book you'll be able to find the right food that better suit you and help you stay healthy.

The next step is to:

- Categorize yourself in terms of your lifestyle.

- Choose the diet that better fits your lifestyle.

- Balance your diet every day in order to get the right nutrients.

- Balance meals on your plates according to the nutrients you bring to your plate.

- Do the appropriate research and find out the number of options you available for you out there.

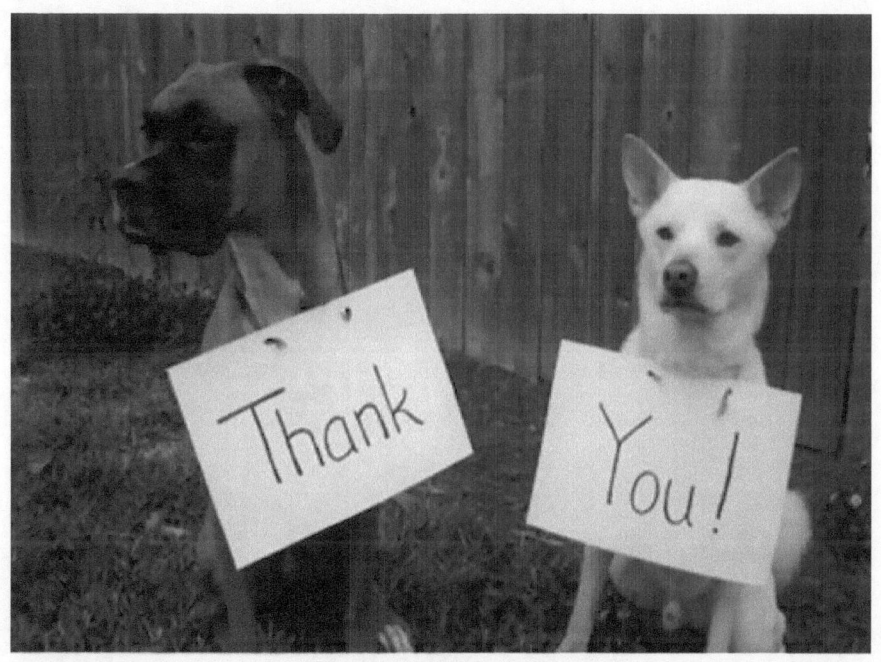

Finally, if you enjoyed this book, then I'd like to ask you for a favor, would you be kind enough to leave a review for this book on Amazon? It'd be greatly appreciated!

Thank you and good luck!